KETO BAKING

Discover 30 Easy to Follow Ketogenic Baking Cookbook recipes for Your Low-Carb Diet with Gluten-Free and wheat to Maximize your weight loss

STEPHANIE BAKER

Copyright © Stephanie Baker

All rights reserved. No part of this book may be reproduced, scanned or distributed in any printed or electronic form without permission. Please do not participate in or encourage piracy of copyrighted materials in violation of the author's rights. Purchase only authorized editions.

1
CINNAMON FLAXSEED KETO CRUNCHY

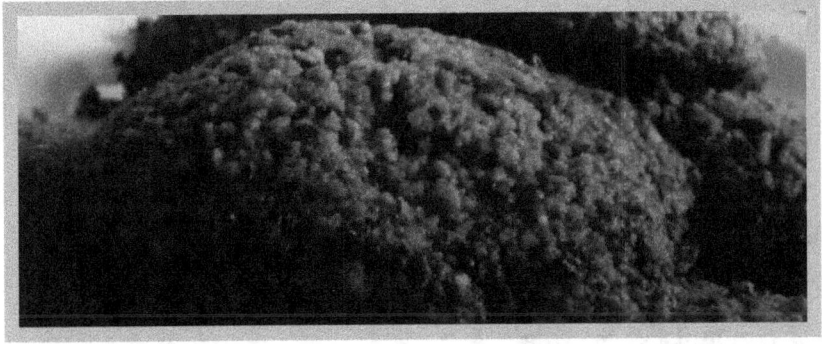

40 MINUTES

Servings: 6

INGREDIENTS

80 g ground almonds

2 teaspoons of cinnamon

30 g ground flaxseed

2 EL Xucker light erythritol

80 g butter

. . .

PREPARATION

Prepare the ingredients for the keto recipe.

Flaxseed Cinnamon Crunchie Recipe LCHF

Preheat the oven to 200°C and line a baking sheet with parchment paper.

Mix the ground almonds, flaxseed flour, cinnamon and xucker in a food processor (alternatively with a hand blender) until it is properly mixed.

Then sprinkle pieces of butter over the mixture and mix again until the dough is roughly crumbly.

Keto Cinnamon Flaxseed Crunchy Recipe

Spread the batter on the baking sheet and bake in the oven for 20 to 25 minutes until the keto chrunchies are golden brown.

After you've let the crunchies cool down (only then will they get nice and crispy), they're ready to serve.

NUTRITION FACTS

Cinnamon Flaxseed Keto Crunchy Recipe
Amount Per Serving
Calories 195Calories from Fat 180
% Daily Value *
Fat 20g31%
Saturated Fat 7g35%
Polyunsaturated Fat 3g
Monounsaturated Fat 3g
Cholesterol 32mg11%
Sodium 2mg0%
Potassium 142mg4%

Carbohydrates 1g 3%
Fiber 4g 16%
Sugar 0.02g 0%
Protein 4g 8th%
Vitamin A 600IU 12%
Vitamin C 0.2mg 0%
Calcium 60mg 6%
Iron 1.6mg 9%
* Percent Daily Valuesare based on a 2000 calorie diet.

2
KETO EASTER BREAD - LOW CARB BREAD

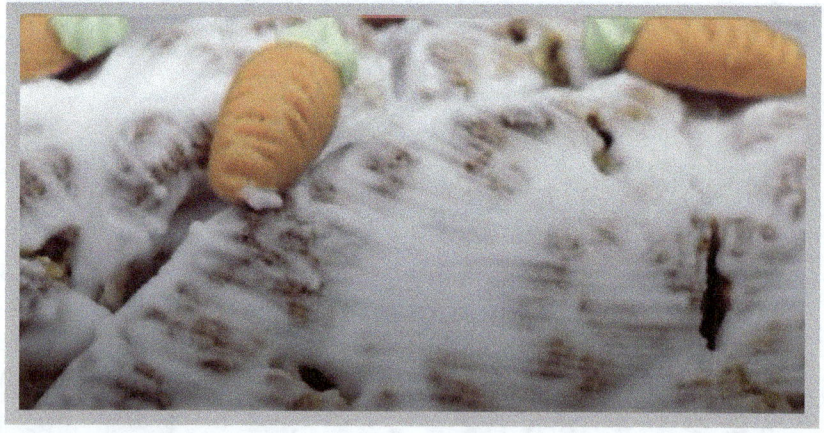

1 HOUR 55 minutes
Servings 15

INGREDIENTS

250 g flax flour
115 g almond flour
35 g coconut flour
200 g eggs
1 packet of dry yeast
1 teaspoon of sugar
300 ml almond milk
2 teaspoons of salt

PREPARATION

Knead all ingredients into a dough with a food processor. Cover and let rise in a warm place for 60 minutes.

Preheat the oven to 160° convection.

Knead the dough well again and place on a baking sheet. Bake at 160° for 40-50 minutes.

Let cool and decorate with a topping if you like.
Nutrition Facts
Keto Easter bread - low carb bread
Amount Per Serving (60 g)
Calories 114Calories from Fat 36
% Daily Value *
Fat 4g6%
Saturated Fat 0.4g2%
Cholesterol 51mg17%
Sodium 15mg1%
Potassium 0.1mg0%
Carbohydrates 2g7%
Fiber 3g12%
Sugar 1g1%

Protein 12g 24%
Vitamin A 100IU 2%
Calcium 10mg 1%
Iron 0.2mg 1%
* Percent Daily Values are based on a 2000 calorie diet.

3
LOW CARB ZUCCHINI BREAD

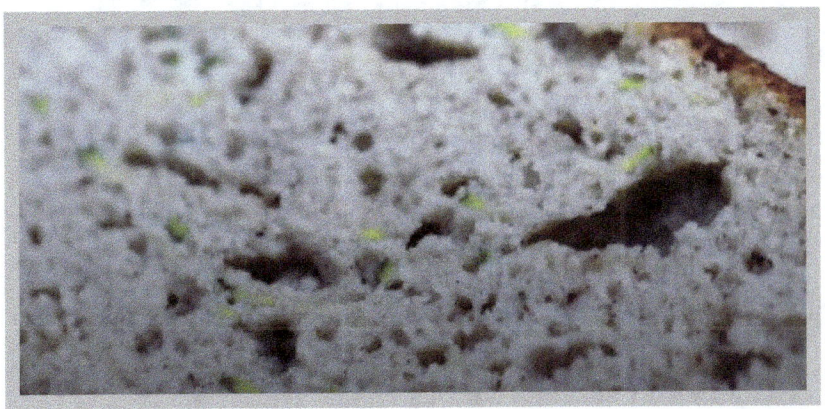

1 HOUR 20 minutes
Servings 18

INGREDIENTS
80 g zucchini
500 g eggs

90 g butter
30 g stevia sweetener
10 g almond butter
80 g coconut flour
1 g baking powder 1 tsp
2 teaspoons of cinnamon
Ground 1/2 teaspoon ginger
1 teaspoon salt
1 teaspoon vanilla extract

PREPARATION

Preheat the oven to 150 ° convection.

Either grease a loaf pan well or line it with baking paper.

Chop the zucchini very finely with a food processor.

Now process all ingredients with the food processor into a smooth dough and fill the loaf pan.

Bake in the oven for about 60 minutes. Let it cool down after taking it out.

Nutrition Facts

Low carb zucchini bread

Amount Per Serving (44 g)

Calories 95Calories from Fat 72

% Daily Value *

Fat 8g12%

Saturated Fat 4g20%

Cholesterol 106mg35%

Sodium 31mg1%

Potassium 0.004mg0%

Carbohydrates 1g3%

Fiber 2g8th%

Sugar 1g1%
Protein 4g8th%
Vitamin A 200IU4%
Calcium 10mg1%
Iron 0.4mg2%
* Percent Daily Valuesare based on a 2000 calorie diet.

4
ALMOND BISCUITS

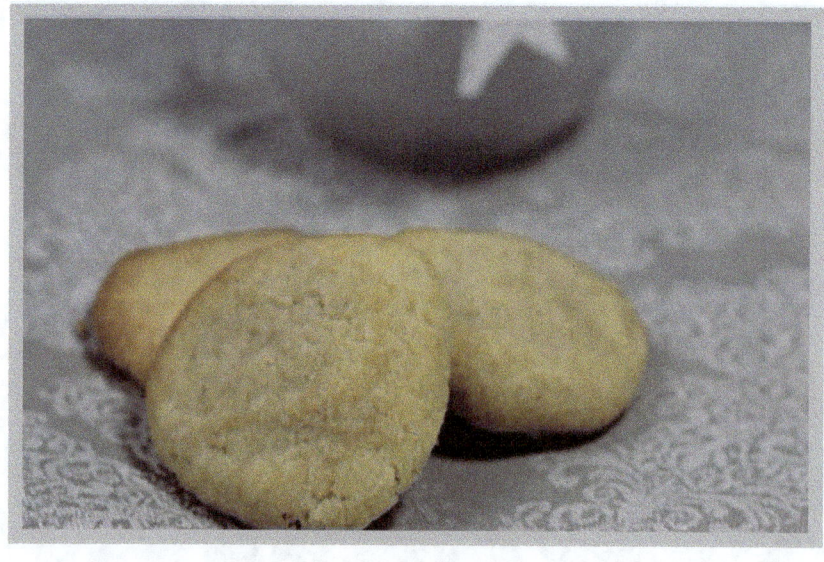

1 HOUR 15 minutes
Servings 20

INGREDIENTS

250 g almond flour
1 egg
10 g stevia extract powder
125 g pasture butter
25 g erythritol powdered sugar
2 ml vanilla flavor
1 pinch of salt

PREPARATION

Have all the ingredients ready for the recipe.
Ingredients for low carb almond biscuits
Mix all ingredients and knead into a biscuit dough.
Bake almond cookies yourself
Chill the dough in the refrigerator for 1 hour.
Almond Cookie Biscuit Dough
Then preheat the oven (150°C, fan oven) and line 2 baking trays with baking paper.
Then roll out the biscuit dough and cut out figures with cookie cutters.
Bake the biscuits for 10 minutes.
Almond Cookies Keto Recipes LCHF
Nutrition Facts
almond biscuits
Amount Per Serving (23 g)
Calories 124Calories from Fat 108
% Daily Value *
Fat 12g18%

Saturated Fat 3g 15%
Polyunsaturated Fat 0.03g
Monounsaturated Fat 0.1g
Cholesterol 24mg 8th%
Sodium 52mg 2%
Potassium 3mg 0%
Carbohydrates 1g 3%
Fiber 1g 4%
Sugar 1g 1%
Protein 3g 6%
Vitamin A 250IU 5%
Calcium 2mg 0%
Iron 0.1mg 1%

* Percent Daily Valuesare based on a 2000 calorie diet.

5
CINNAMON STARS

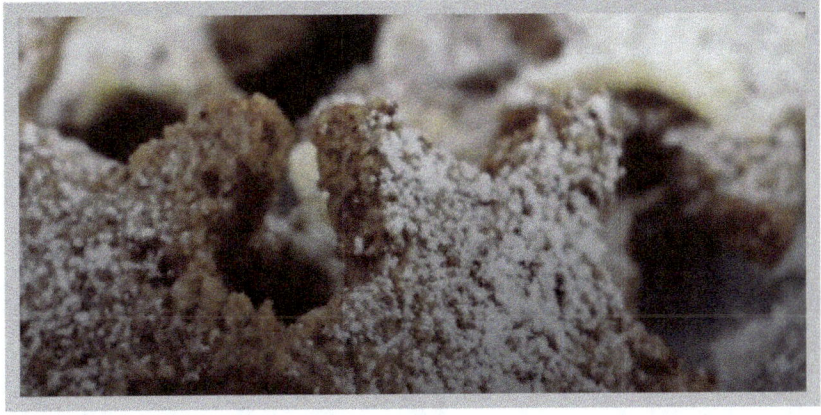

30 MINUTES
Servings 8

INGREDIENTS
100 g ground hazelnuts
100 g ground almonds

2 eggs
1 pinch of salt
1 teaspoon lemon juice
80 g of erythritol
1 teaspoon ground vanilla
3 teaspoons of cinnamon

PREPARATION

Prepare all the ingredients for the recipe
Low carb cinnamon star recipe ketogenic
Beat the eggs, separate the egg white from the yolk and beat the egg white until stiff. Set aside 3 tbsp.

Knead the remaining ingredients into a dough with a food processor.
Making cinnamon star dough Ketofix
Preheat the oven (160°C). Roll out the cookie dough about 1cm thick and cut out stars with a cookie cutter.
Cinnamon star dough recipes ketogenic diet
Spread the stars on a baking sheet ...
Keto Zimtsterne Low-Carb Recipes
... and brush with the egg whites that have been set aside.
Bake Christmas cookies Zimtsterne low-carb
Bake in the oven for about 10 minutes at 160°C (fan oven).
Enjoy the cinnamon stars!
RECIPE NOTES
1 serving corresponds to 3 - 4 cinnamon stars

. . .

Nutrition Facts

Cinnamon stars

Amount Per Serving (50 g)

Calories 178 Calories from Fat 144

% Daily Value *

Fat 16g 25%

Saturated Fat 0.4g 2%

Polyunsaturated Fat 1g

Monounsaturated Fat 0.5g

Cholesterol 53mg 18%

Sodium 18mg 1%

Potassium 121mg 3%

Carbohydrates 2g 7%

Fiber 3g 12%

Sugar 0.2g 0%

Protein 5g 10%

Vitamin A 100IU 2%

Vitamin C 0.1mg 0%

Calcium 40mg 4%

Iron 0.9mg 5%

* Percent Daily Valuesare based on a 2000 calorie diet.

6
LOW CARB KETO MUFFIN BUNS

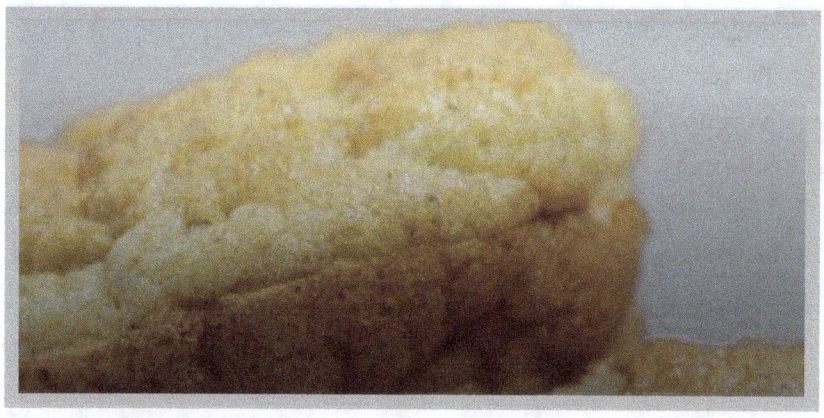

30 MINUTES
Servings 12

INGREDIENTS
150 g eggs

60 g cream cheese
15 g psyllium husks
10 g coconut flour

PREPARATION

Preheat the oven to 150 ° convection.

Separate the eggs and beat the egg whites very stiff.

Mix the egg yolk with the remaining ingredients and carefully fold into the egg whites.

Now fill the dough into twelve muffin molds and bake in the oven for about 20 minutes.

You can conjure up these mini burgers with the Keto Muffin Buns.

Nutrition Facts

Low carb keto muffin buns

Amount Per Serving (19 g)

Calories 33Calories from Fat 18

% Daily Value *

Fat 2g3%

Saturated Fat 0.4g2%

Cholesterol 48mg16%

Sodium 14mg1%

Carbohydrates 0.4g1%

Fiber 0.3g1%

Sugar 0.2g0%

Protein 2g 4%
Vitamin A 100IU 2%
Calcium 10mg 1%
Iron 0.2mg 1%
* Percent Daily Values are based on a 2000 calorie diet.

7
5 MINUTE MICRO LOW CARB BREAD

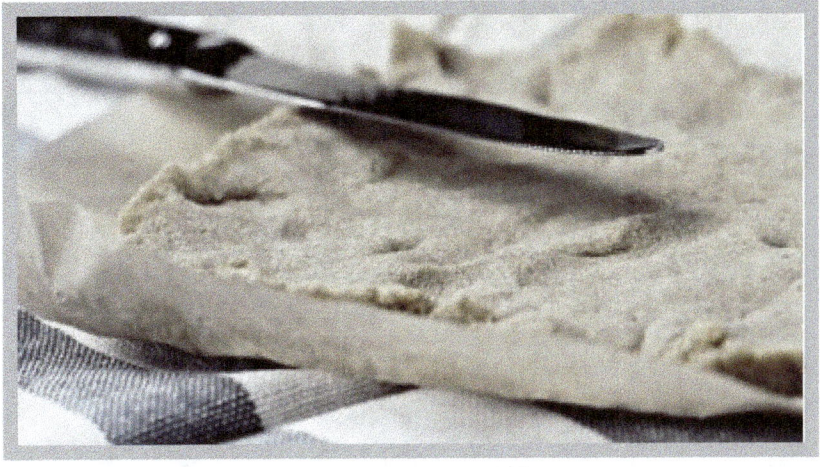

5 MINUTES

Servings 2

INGREDIENTS

30 g almond flour
20 g low carb potato fiber
30 g butter
1 egg
1 pinch of salt

PREPARATION

Prepare the ingredients for the low carb bread
Low carb bread recipe ingredients
Melt the butter
Mix all ingredients together to form a dough
Press the bread dough into a mold
Bake the low carb bread in the microwave for 2 minutes on the highest setting
Your micro low carb bread is now ready to serve
Nutrition Facts
Amount Per Serving (65 g)
Calories 259Calories from Fat 207
% Daily Value *
Fat 23g35%
Saturated Fat 8g40%
Polyunsaturated Fat 1g
Monounsaturated Fat 5g
Cholesterol 142mg47%
Sodium 40mg2%
Potassium 36mg1%
Carbohydrates 2g7%
Fiber 8g32%
Sugar 1g1%
Protein 7g14%

Vitamin A 750IU 15%
Vitamin C 0mg 0%
Calcium 20mg 2%
Iron 0.5mg 3%
* Percent Daily Values are based on a 2000 calorie diet.

8
LOW CARB KETO BREAKFAST CAKE

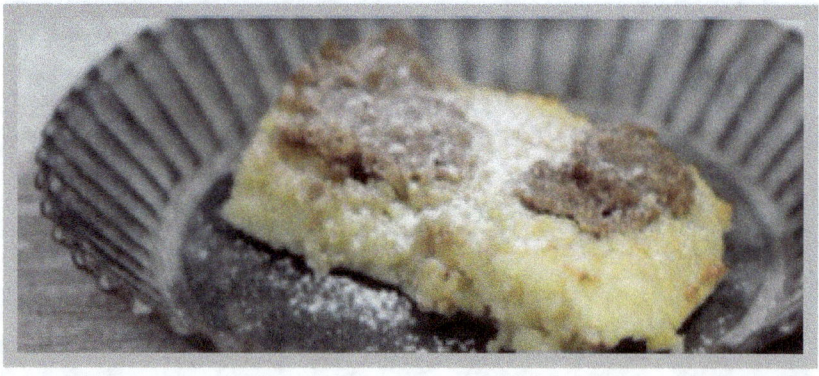

50 MINUTES
Servings 4

INGREDIENTS
SPRINKLES
20 g almond flour
20 g stevia sugar

3 ml coconut oil
1/2 teaspoon cinnamon
GROUND
120 g almond flour
90 g Greek yogurt
80 g stevia powder
50 g egg
1 teaspoon vanilla extract

PREPARATION

Preheat the oven to 150 ° convection.

Grease a small baking pan (ø 18 cm) or line it with baking paper.

For the crumble, work all the ingredients into a dough with your hands and set it aside.

Mix all ingredients for the base with a food processor and pour into the mold.

Spread the streusel on top and bake in the oven for about 20 minutes.

Nutrition Facts

Amount Per Serving (90 g)

Calories 186Calories from Fat 72

% Daily Value *

Fat 8g12%

Saturated Fat 3g15%

Polyunsaturated Fat 0.2g

Monounsaturated Fat 1g

Cholesterol 53mg18%

Sodium 18mg1%

Potassium 17mg0%

Carbohydrates 5g17%
Fiber 8g32%
Sugar 5g6%
Protein 18g36%
Vitamin A 50IU1%
Calcium 10mg1%
Iron 0.2mg1%
* Percent Daily Valuesare based on a 2000 calorie diet.

9
LOW CARB KETO BREAD "SOUL BREAD"

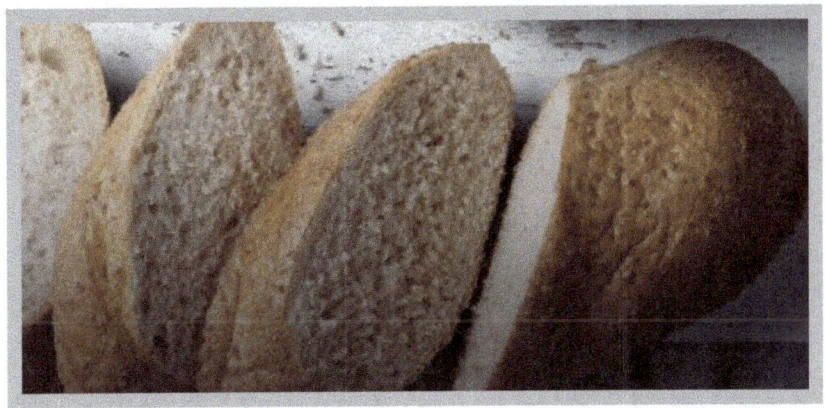

1 HOUR 5 minutes
Servings 15

INGREDIENTS
250 g cream cheese
30 g butter

45 ml of olive oil

45 ml of cream

4 pieces of eggs

1 teaspoon baking soda

3 tsp psyllium husks

1/2 teaspoon salt

90 g whey protein powder neutral

5 drops of stevia liquid

PREPARATION

Put together the ingredients for the low carb keto bread "Soul Bread".

Low Carb Keto Diet Bread Recipe

Preheat the oven to 180°C (fan-assisted) and line a baking pan with baking paper.

Put all ingredients in a large bowl and knead into a dough with a Kitchen Aid (if available).

Pour the bread dough into the baking pan and bake in the oven for 50 minutes.

Then take the bread out of the oven and let it cool for 10 minutes before taking it out of the baking pan.

Your self-baked low carb keto "Soul Bread" is ready.

Low carb keto bread soul bread

RECIPE NOTES

Tip: Try the bread straight with butter. It tastes great. A large part of our food is eaten this way. It is also a pleasure with our keto jam and low carb jam. Of course, you can also put sausage or cheese on the keto bread. Everyone can enjoy it in their own way.

. . .

Nutrition Facts

Low Carb Keto Bread "Soul Bread"

Amount Per Serving

Calories 133 Calories from Fat 81

% Daily Value *

Fat 9g 14%

Saturated Fat 6g 30%

Polyunsaturated Fat 1g

Monounsaturated Fat 5g

Cholesterol 23mg 8th%

Sodium 140mg 6%

Potassium 23mg 1%

Carbohydrates 1g 3%

Fiber 1g 4%

Sugar 0.4g 0%

Protein 6g 12%

Vitamin A 350IU 7%

Vitamin C 0mg 0%

Calcium 20mg 2%

Iron 0.2mg 1%

* Percent Daily Valuesare based on a 2000 calorie diet.

10
KETO PANCAKES

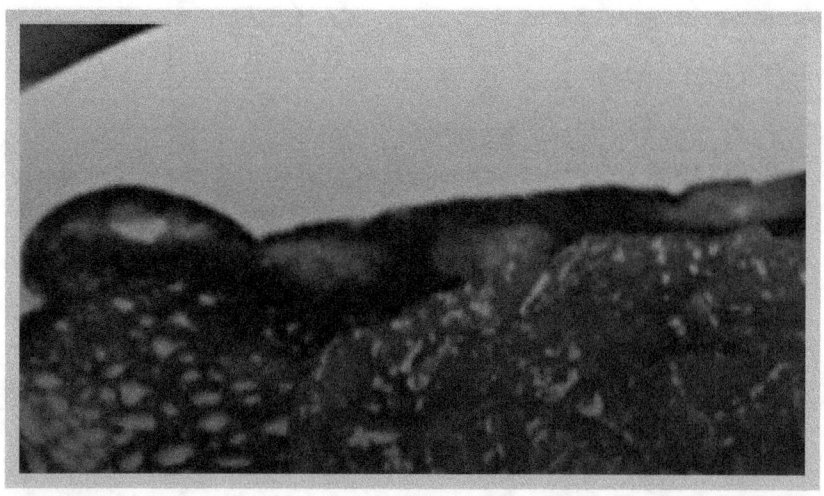

13 MINUTES
 Servings 2

. . .

INGREDIENTS

3 eggs
80 g cream cheese

PREPARATION

Mix the egg and cream cheese batter (if available in a food processor)

Bake in a pan (yield: 12 small pancakes)

Use low carb applesauce as a topping for serving

RECIPE NOTES

To increase the fat content, brush the pancakes with plenty of butter, for example.

NUTRITION FACTS

Keto pancakes

Amount Per Serving (115 g)

Calories 251Calories from Fat 153

% Daily Value *

Fat 17g26%

Saturated Fat 2g10%

Polyunsaturated Fat 1g

Monounsaturated Fat 3g

Cholesterol 362mg121%

Sodium 223mg9%

Potassium 148mg4%

Carbohydrates 2g7%

Sugar 2g 2%
Protein 12g 24%
Vitamin A 900IU 18%
Calcium 80mg 8th%
Iron 1.8mg 10%
* Percent Daily Values are based on a 2000 calorie diet.

11
KETO CHOCOLATE CHEESECAKE CHOCOLATE CAKE

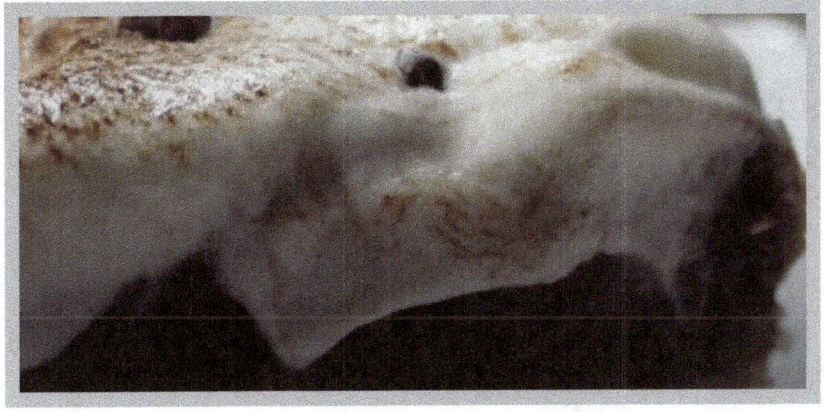

45 MINUTES
Servings 12

INGREDIENTS
CAKE BASE
300 g ground hazelnuts

60 g butter (soft)

3 teaspoons of erythritol

1 pinch of salt

CAKE TOPPING

400 g mascarpone

200 g dark chocolate 99% cocoa

6 teaspoons of erythritol

70 g butter (soft)

50 ml of cream

TOPPING

150 ml of cream

DECO / REFINE

Cocoa nibs

Cocoa powder

PREPARATION

Put all the ingredients for the cake recipe together and preheat the oven (180° C, fan oven)

Chocolate Cake Cheesecake Ingredients

CAKE BASE

Mix the butter, the ground hazelnuts, salt and erythritol together and knead a cake batter

Line a 24 cm springform pan with parchment paper

Spread the dough evenly in the mold, press it flat and form a 1cm high rim

Cheesecake cake base recipe

Bake the cake base in the oven for 15 minutes

CAKE TOPPING PREPARATION WITH THE COOKING CHEF FOOD PROCESSOR

Heat all the ingredients for the cake topping at 40°C in the

Cooking Chef ...

Melting chocolate by Kenwood Cooking Chef

... and mix

Kenwood Cooking Chef Melting Chocolate

CAKE TOPPING PREPARATION WITHOUT A COOKING CHEF

Heat and liquefy the mascarpone

Melt the chocolate in a double boiler

Mix the remaining cake topping ingredients with the mascarpone and chocolate

COMPLETE

Spread the mixture on the cake and chill the chocolate cheesecake in the refrigerator for 2 hours

Low-carb chocolate cake recipe

Then whip the cream for the topping until stiff and spread on the chocolate cake

Refine with cocoa powder and cocoa nibs and serve

Chocolate Cheesecake Chocolate Cake Ketofix

Nutrition Facts

Keto Chocolate Cheesecake Chocolate Cake

Amount Per Serving (105 g)

Calories 520 Calories from Fat 459

% Daily Value *

Fat 51g 78%

Saturated Fat 15g 75%

Polyunsaturated Fat 2g

Monounsaturated Fat 16g

Cholesterol 28mg 9%

Sodium 46mg 2%

Potassium 215mg 6%

Carbohydrates 5g 17%

Fiber 3g 12%
Sugar 2g 2%
Protein 8g 16%
Vitamin A 800IU 16%
Vitamin C 2.5mg 3%
Calcium 40mg 4%
Iron 1.3mg 7%
* Percent Daily Values are based on a 2000 calorie diet.

12
LOW CARB CARROT CAKE CARROT CAKE RECIPE

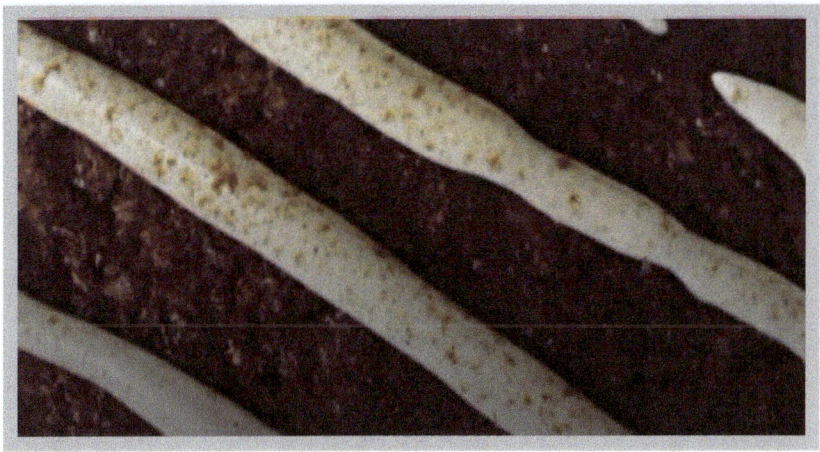

50 MINUTES

Servings 12

INGREDIENTS

5 eggs

200 g carrots
200 g butter
170 g cream cheese
100 g almond flour
30 g walnuts chopped
20 g desiccated coconut
4 tbsp erythritol
2 teaspoons of baking powder
1 teaspoon ground cinnamon
1 bottle of vanilla flavor

PREPARATION

Put together the ingredients for the carrot cake

Carrot cake baking ingredients

Preheat the oven to 180° C (convection)

Grate the carrots

Mix eggs, butter, 1 tbsp erythritol and vanilla flavor into a dough

Low-carb carrot cake baking recipes

Add the grated carrots, walnuts, almond flour, baking powder and desiccated coconut and mix well

Bake carrot cakes yourself

Pour the cake batter into a baking pan and bake for about 40 minutes

Then let it cool down

Heat the cream cheese in the microwave for 20 seconds on medium power

Mix the cream cheese with the remaining erythritol and spread over the cake

Finally, garnish the carrot cake with cinnamon

. . .

NUTRITION FACTS

Low carb carrot cake carrot cake recipe
Amount Per Serving (85 g)
Calories 290 Calories from Fat 234
% Daily Value *
Fat 26g 40%
Saturated Fat 10g 50%
Polyunsaturated Fat 2g
Monounsaturated Fat 5g
Cholesterol 144mg 48%
Sodium 174mg 7%
Potassium 112mg 3%
Carbohydrates 3g 10%
Fiber 2g 8th%
Sugar 2g 2%
Protein 6g 12%
Vitamin A 3800IU 76%
Vitamin C 1.7mg 2%
Calcium 80mg 8th%
Iron 0.9mg 5%
* Percent Daily Valuesare based on a 2000 calorie diet.

13
LOW CARB KETO WAFFLE RECIPE JALAPENO CHEDDAR

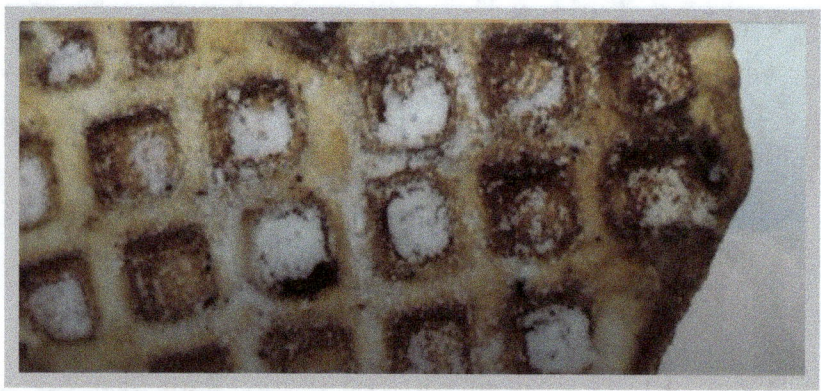

10 MINUTES
SERVINGS 2

INGREDIENTS
80 g cream cheese
3 eggs

1 EL coconut flour
1 teaspoon flea seed husks
1 teaspoon baking powder
30 grams of cheddar
1 jalapeno
salt
pepper

INSTRUCTIONS

Put all the ingredients in a bowl.

Mix them with a hand blender until the mixture has turned into an evenly fine waffle batter.

Turn on the waffle iron.

As soon as the waffle iron is hot enough, pour the waffle batter into it.

Remove the low carb waffle when it's the right consistency for your taste.

Now you can serve the waffle.

RECIPE NOTES

Low Carb High Fat (LCHF) and suitable for the ketogenic diet.

NUTRITION FACTS

Low Carb Keto Waffle Recipe Jalapeno Cheddar

Amount Per Serving (130 g)

Calories 340 Calories from Fat 198

% Daily Value *

Fat 22g 34%
Saturated Fat 5g 25%
Polyunsaturated Fat 1g
Monounsaturated Fat 4g
Cholesterol 378mg 126%
Sodium 578mg 24%
Potassium 178mg 5%
Carbohydrates 4g 13%
Fiber 4g 16%
Sugar 3g 3%
Protein 17g 34%
Vitamin A 1100IU 22%
Vitamin C 4.1mg 5%
Calcium 330mg 33%
Iron 2.3mg 13%
* Percent Daily Valuesare based on a 2000 calorie diet.

14
KETO CURD CREPES RECIPE

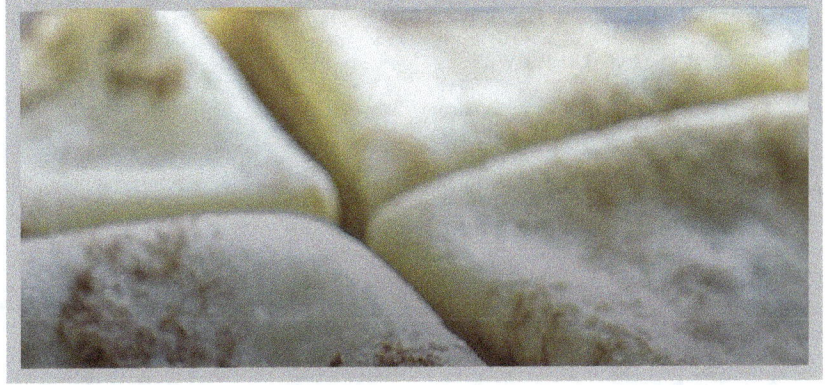

16 MINUTES
Servings 3

INGREDIENTS
100 g quark 40% fat
3 eggs

15 g erythritol

PREPARATION

Preheat the oven to 150°C (fan oven) and prepare a baking sheet with baking paper.

Put the quark, eggs and erythritol in a bowl and stir with a whisk.

Spread the crepes batter on the baking sheet and bake for 10 minutes in the oven.

Cut the dough into small portions and enjoy for breakfast.

RECIPE NOTES

Low Carb Recipe for the Ketogenic Diet . Also suitable for cold eating and to take away.

Nutrition Facts

Amount Per Serving (265 g)
Calories 122Calories from Fat 81
% Daily Value *
Fat 9g14%
Saturated Fat 2g10%
Polyunsaturated Fat 1g
Monounsaturated Fat 2g
Cholesterol 222mg74%
Sodium 70mg3%
Potassium 67mg2%
Carbohydrates 1g3%
Sugar 1g1%

Protein 10g 20%
Vitamin A 250IU 5%
Calcium 30mg 3%
Iron 0.9mg 5%
* Percent Daily Values are based on a 2000 calorie diet.

15

PEANUT BUTTER KETO COOKIES RECIPE

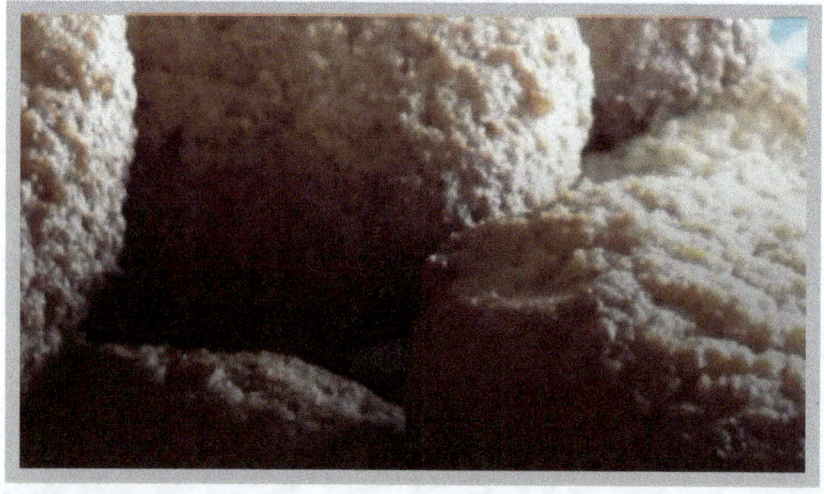

30 MINUTES
Servings 15

INGREDIENTS

100 g peanut butter
1 egg
45 g Xucker light (erythritol)
25 g coconut flour
13 g psyllium husks
70 g butter
10 g cream
1 teaspoon baking powder
1/4 teaspoon baking soda

PREPARATION

Put together all the ingredients for the keto recipe.
Recipes Diet Biscuits LCHF
Preheat the oven to 180°C (fan-assisted) and prepare a baking sheet with baking paper.
Mix all ingredients with the Kitchen Aid to form a dough.
Keto Diet Cookies Recipe
Shape the cookie dough into small balls with your hands, place them on the baking paper and flatten them a little.
Peanut Butter Keto Cookies Recipe LCHF
Put in the oven and finish baking for 10 minutes.
Then let it cool down until the peanut butter keto cookies are ready to serve.

Nutrition Facts
Amount Per Serving
Calories 84Calories from Fat 63
% Daily Value *
Fat 7g11%

Saturated Fat 2g 10%
Polyunsaturated Fat 0.1g
Monounsaturated Fat 1g
Cholesterol 11mg 4%
Sodium 58mg 2%
Potassium 1mg 0%
Carbohydrates 1g 3%
Fiber 2g 8th%
Sugar 1g 1%
Protein 2g 4%
Vitamin A 200IU 4%
Vitamin C 0mg 0%
Calcium 20mg 2%
Iron 0mg 0%
* Percent Daily Valuesare based on a 2000 calorie diet.

16

KETO CHEESY RANCH CHICKEN AND CAULIFLOWER RICE

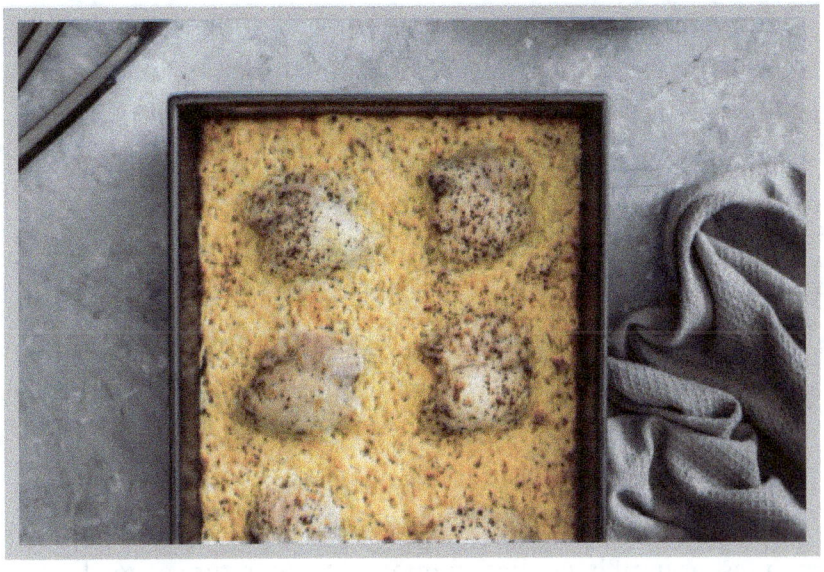

55 MINUTES

Servings 4

. . .

INSTRUCTION

- 2 tablespoon butter
- 4 ounce cream cheese
- 4 tablespoon ranch dressing
- 20 ounce cauliflower rice
- 1/2 cup shredded cheddar cheese
- 24 ounce boneless + skinless chicken thighs
- 1 tablespoon olive oil
- Salt and pepper to taste

PREPARATION

Both ingredients should be measured out and ready to use. Preheat the oven to 375 degrees Fahrenheit.

Combine butter, cream cheese, and half of the ranch dressing in a microwave-safe dish. Microwave for 1 minute, or until fully melted.

To the melted mixture, add the cauliflower rice and shredded cheddar cheese. To taste, season with salt and pepper.

Spread the cauliflower rice mixture out flat in a baking dish with a spatula.

Toss the chicken with the remaining ranch dressing and season with salt and pepper to taste. In a baking dish, place the seasoned chicken.

Drizzle with extra virgin olive oil.

Preheat the oven to 400°F and bake the chicken for 40-45 minutes, or until it reaches an internal temperature of 165°F.

Allow for a few minutes of cooling before serving. Have fun!

17
KETO FISH CASSEROLE

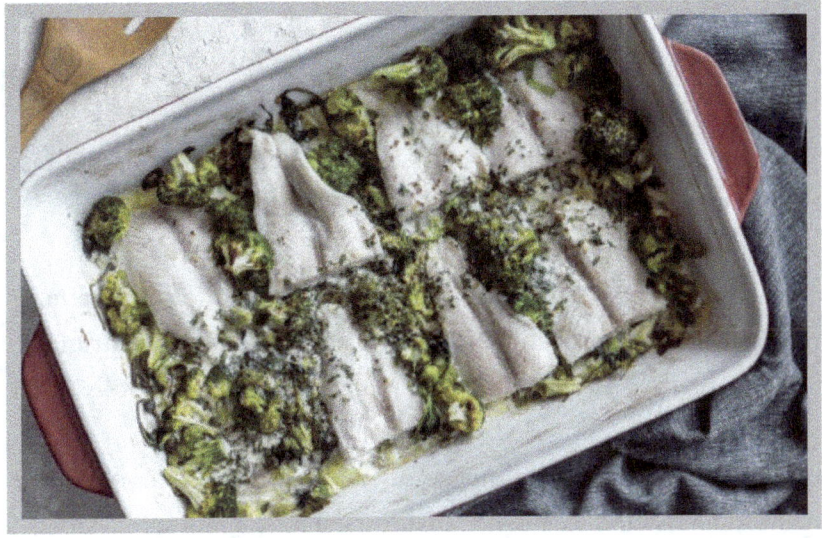

45 MINUTES
Servings 4

. . .

INSTRUCTIONS

2 tablespoon olive oil

16 ounce broccoli

5 ounce spinach

6 medium green onion

2 tablespoon capers

1 tablespoon butter, for greasing dish

24 ounce white fish

1 1/4 cup heavy cream

1/2 medium lemon, juice of

1 tablespoon dijon mustard

1 tablespoon fresh parsley, chopped

6 tablespoon butter

Salt and pepper to taste

PREPARATION

All ingredients should be measured and prepared. Preheat the oven to 400 degrees Fahrenheit and butter a baking dish.

Broccoli stems should be held and cut into small florets.

In a medium-sized pan, heat the oil. When the pan is warmed, add the broccoli and cook for 4-5 minutes, or until fork-tender. Enable the broccoli to wilt for 45-60 seconds after adding the spinach.

Apply the green onions and capers to the pan once the spinach has wilted. Cook for an additional 1-2 minutes.

Place the vegetables in the baking dish that has been greased. Place the fish on top of the vegetables, with the vegetables covering the sides of the fish.

Combine the heavy cream, lemon juice, Dijon mustard, and

chopped parsley in a large mixing bowl. Pour the sauce over the fish and vegetables, then finish with butter slices. Bake for 20 minutes, or until the fish is flaky.

Heat it up and enjoy it!

18

KETO CHICKEN PHILLY CHEESESTEAK

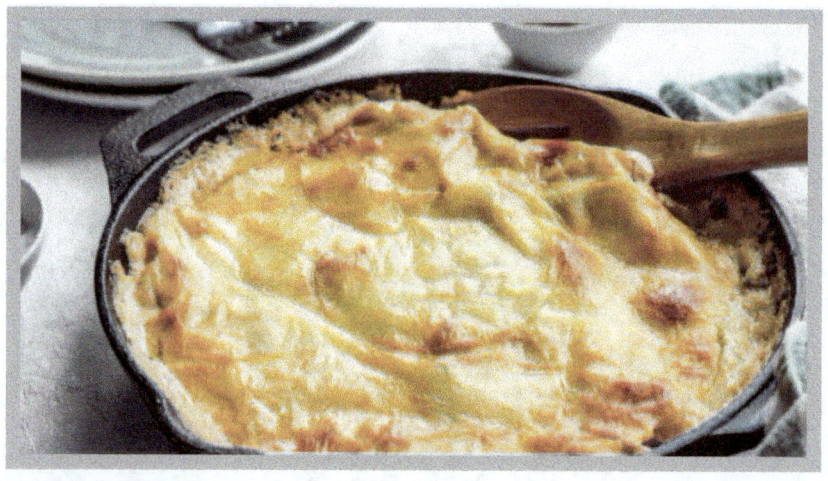

1 HOUR

Servings 8

INGREDIENTS

- 1 tablespoon butter
- 32 ounce boneless chicken thighs, diced
- 1/2 medium yellow onion, chopped
- 1 medium green bell pepper, sliced
- 8 ounce cremini mushrooms, halved
- 2 teaspoon fresh garlic
- Salt and pepper to taste
- 8 ounce cream cheese, softened
- 1/2 cup heavy cream
- 2 tablespoon worcestershire sauce
- 8 ounce cheddar cheese, shredded
- 8 ounce provolone cheese

PREPARATION

Both ingredients should be measured out and ready to use. Preheat the oven to 375 degrees Fahrenheit.

In a frying pan, melt butter over medium to high heat. Fry the chicken until it is finished.

Add the onion, bell pepper, and mushrooms after that. Add half of the garlic and season to taste with salt and pepper. Cook the chicken and vegetables in a skillet until they are tender. Then turn off the heat.

Combine the remaining garlic cloves, cream cheese, heavy cream, Worcestershire sauce, and shredded cheddar cheese in a mixing bowl. Combine the chicken and vegetables in a mixing bowl.

Serve in a baking dish with provolone cheese on top.

Preheat the oven to 350°F and bake for 25-30 minutes, or until the cheese is golden brown. Have fun!

KETO BAKED CAESAR CHICKEN

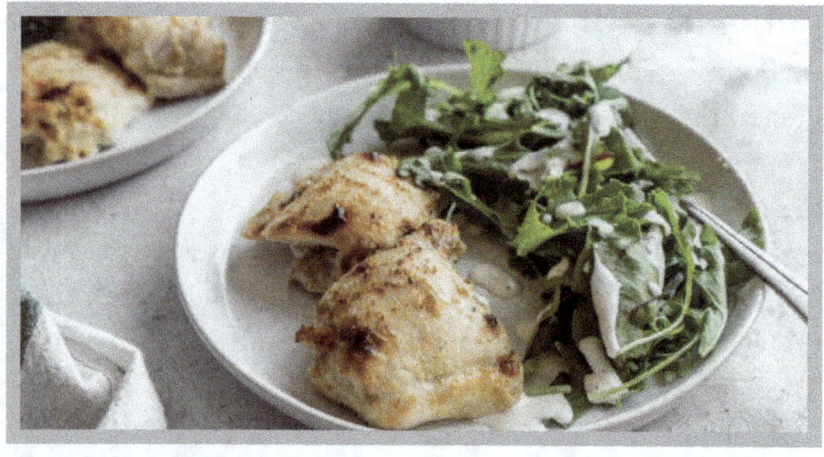

2 HOURS, 40 minutes
Servings 2

INGREDIENTS

12 ounce boneless, skinless chicken thighs

4 tablespoon caesar dressing
1 teaspoon lemon juice
1 teaspoon kosher salt
1/4 teaspoon garlic powder
1/4 teaspoon onion powder
12 ounce spring mix
4 tablespoon caesar dressing

PREPARATION

All of the ingredients should be measured out and ready to use.

Combine the caesar dressing, lemon juice, salt, garlic powder, and onion powder in a mixing bowl. Stir until it is well blended.

Place the chicken in the bowl, smothering it with the marinade and coating every part of it.

Refrigerate for at least 2 hours, but up to 24 hours, after covering with plastic wrap.

Preheat the oven to 400 degrees Fahrenheit before beginning to cook. Arrange the chicken on a baking sheet lined with aluminum foil in an even layer.

Preheat oven to 350°F and bake chicken for 30-35 minutes, or until internal temperature reaches 165°F.

Serve the chicken with more caesar dressing and leafy greens on the side. Have fun!

20

KETO ASPARAGUS WALNUT SALAD

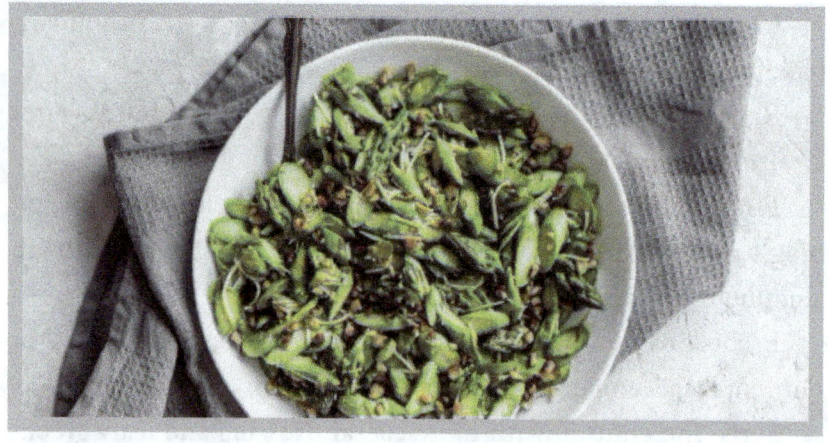

25 MINUTES
Servings 4

INGREDIENTS

1/2 cup walnuts, chopped

- 20 ounce asparagus spears
- 1 medium lemon, juice + zest
- 2 teaspoon chili-garlic paste
- 1 teaspoon salt
- 1/4 cup avocado oil
- 1/2 cup grated parmesan cheese

PREPARATION

All of the ingredients should be measured and prepared. Preheat the oven to 350 degrees Fahrenheit.

Using parchment paper, line a baking sheet. Place the walnuts on the baking sheet, chopped. Bake for about 10 minutes, or until a light golden brown color is achieved.

Remove the fibrous ends of the asparagus spears and wash them (discard the fibrous parts). The asparagus spears should then be thinly sliced at an angle.

Combine the lemon juice, lemon zest, chili garlic paste, salt, and avocado oil in a mixing bowl.

Stir in the grated parmesan cheese until it is well mixed.

Arrange the cut asparagus spears and toasted walnuts on a tray.

Serve with a quick tossing of the dressing on top. Have fun!

21

KETO CHICKEN CAPRESE CASSEROLE

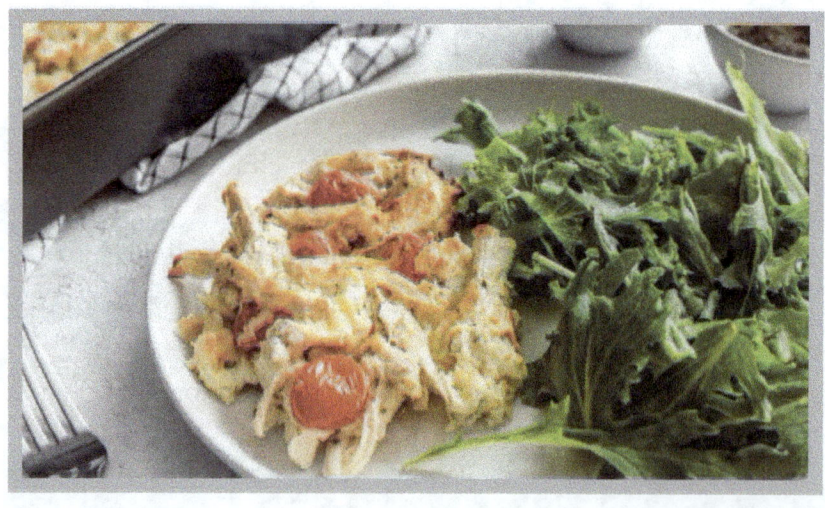

30 MINUTES
Servings 4

INGREDIENTS

20 ounce cooked chicken

7 ounce cherry tomatoes, sliced

8 ounce mozzarella cheese

2 tablespoon pesto

1/2 cup sour cream

1/4 cup mayonnaise

2 ounce parmesan cheese

Salt and pepper to taste

7 ounce leafy greens

1 tablespoon apple cider vinegar

4 tablespoon olive oil

PREPARATION

All of the ingredients should be measured out and ready to use. Preheat the oven to 400 degrees Fahrenheit.

Using a knife, shred the chicken.

The mozzarella cheese should be sliced into small pieces. In a baking dish, mix the shredded chicken, cherry tomatoes, and mozzarella cheese.

Combine pesto, sour cream, mayonnaise, and half of the parmesan cheese in a mixing bowl. Stir until it is well blended. Season to taste with salt and pepper.

Combine this mixture with the ham, onions, and mozzarella cheese in a baking dish. The remaining parmesan cheese should be spread on top. Preheat the oven to 200°F and bake for 20 minutes, or until golden brown.

Toss the leafy greens with apple cider vinegar and serve with a drizzle of olive oil on top as it bakes.

Place the casserole on a plate next to the rice.

22
KETO CREAMY CABBAGE CASSEROLE

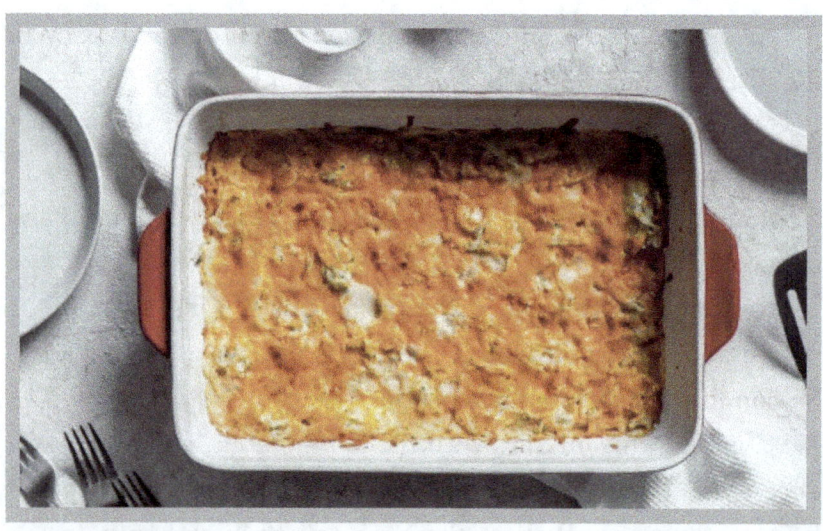

50 MINUTES
Serving 6

. . .

INGREDIENTS

- 8 tablespoon butter
- 32 ounce green cabbage
- 1 medium yellow onion
- 2 teaspoon garlic, minced
- 1 1/2 cup heavy whipping cream
- 6 tablespoon ranch dressing
- 6 ounce cream cheese
- Salt and pepper to taste
- 6 ounce cheddar cheese, shredded

PREPARATION

All of the ingredients should be measured out and ready to use. Preheat the oven to 400 degrees Fahrenheit and grease a baking dish.

Shred the cabbage, onion, and garlic with a mandolin or a sharp knife.

Melt the butter in a frying pan over medium to high heat. Cook for 7-10 minutes, or until the shredded cabbage, onion, and garlic are softened. Combine the heavy cream, ranch dressing, and cream cheese in a mixing bowl. Season to taste with salt and pepper. Stir all together and cook for another 5-8 minutes.

Fill a greased baking pan halfway with the cabbage mixture. Evenly sprinkle the shredded cheddar cheese on top. Bake for 15-20 minutes, or until the cheese has melted and turned golden brown.

SERVE IMMEDIATELY AND ENJOY!

23
KETO LEMON DONUT HOLES

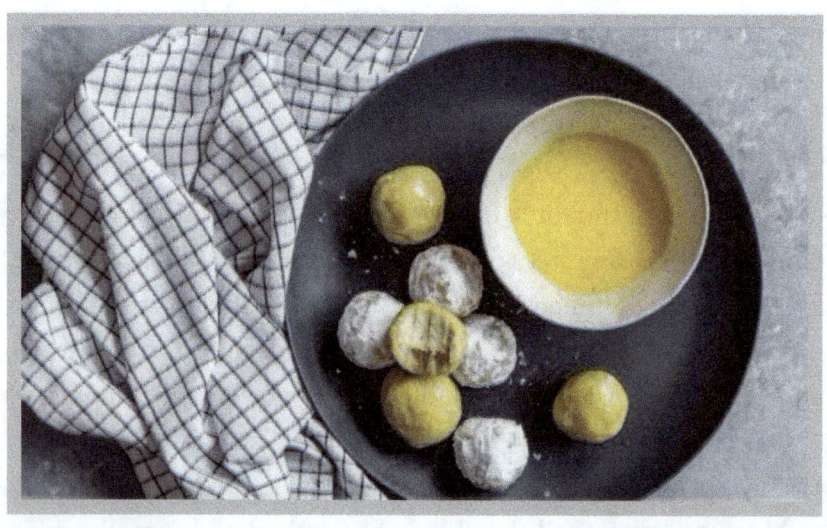

15 MINUTES
Servings 15

. . .

INGREDIENTS

For Donut Holes:

1/2 medium lemon

2 tablespoon avocado oil

1 tablespoon water

1/2 teaspoon vanilla extract

1 cup almond flour

3 tablespoon stevia/erythritol blend

Pinch of salt

For Lemon Glaze:

4 tablespoons powdered stevia/erythritol blend

2 teaspoons lemon juice, as needed

PREPARATION

All of the ingredients should be measured out and ready to use. Preheat the oven to 350 degrees Fahrenheit.

Using parchment paper, line a baking sheet.

Remove the seeds from the lemon and cut it into small wedges.

In a blender, combine the lemon wedges, avocado oil, water, and vanilla extract. Blend on medium until smooth, then strain out any tiny chunks that won't blend.

Combine the almond flour, stevia/erythritol combination, and salt in a mixing bowl. Blend until the mixture has thickened and dough has formed.

Shape balls with a cookie scooper or a dinner spoon and roll with your hands until smooth. Place these on a baking sheet lined with parchment paper. Preheat the oven to 350°F and bake for 10-12 minutes. To make the glaze, combine powdered stevia/erythritol blend and lemon juice in a mixing bowl. Slowly drizzle in the lemon juice, stirring constantly until a smooth glaze forms. Add yellow food coloring to the glaze if desired.

Allow the donuts to cool after they have been removed from the oven.

The lemon glaze should be dipped into the donut holes. You can begin serving immediately

24
KETO CHICKEN CASSEROLE

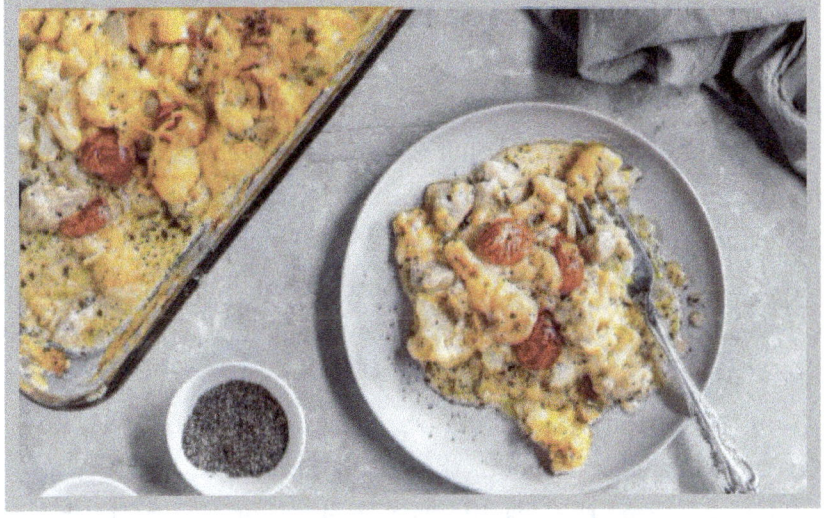

1 HOUR
Servings 6

. . .

INGREDIENTS

- 3/4 cup heavy whipping cream
- 4 ounce cream cheese
- 3 tablespoon pesto
- 1/2 medium lemon, juice of
- Salt and pepper, to taste
- 3 tablespoon butter
- 32 ounce boneless, skinless chicken thighs, cut into pieces
- 1/2 medium yellow onion
- 4 ounce cherry tomatoes, sliced in halves
- 16 ounce cauliflower
- 7 ounce cheddar cheese, shredded

PREPARATION

All ingredients should be gathered and prepared. Preheat the oven to 400 degrees Fahrenheit.

Combine strong whipping cream, cream cheese, pesto, and lemon juice in a mixing bowl. Season with salt and pepper to taste and stir until well mixed.

Melt the butter in a frying pan over medium to high heat. Cook until the cut up chicken pieces are golden brown in color in the pan.

In the bottom of a baking pan, position the cooked chicken. On top of the chicken, pour the cream mixture.

Finish with the cauliflower, yellow onion, and cherry tomatoes.

Add shredded cheddar cheese on top of it. Bake for 25-30 minutes, or until cheese has melted and cauliflower is completely cooked.

Serve and have fun!

25
KETO COCONUT PECAN CHIA BARS

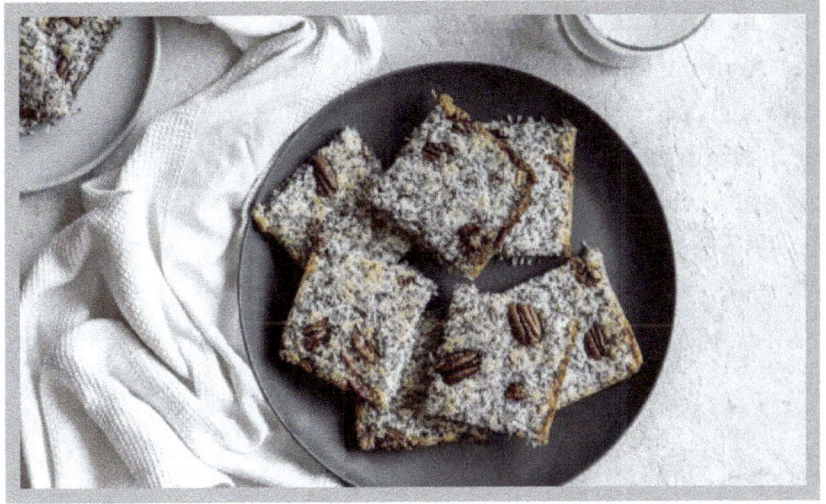

1 HOUR, 5 minutes
Servings 4

. . .

INGREDIENTS

- 4 tablespoon chia seeds
- 1/2 cup water
- 1 cup unsweetened shredded coconut
- 1 tablespoon coconut oil
- 1 tablespoon powdered stevia/erythritol blend
- 1/4 teaspoon vanilla extract
- 1/2 cup pecans

PREPARATION

All ingredients should be gathered and prepared. Preheat the oven to 350 degrees Fahrenheit.

Combine the chia seeds and water in a bowl and set aside for 15 minutes, or until it thickens.

Combine the soaked chia seeds, unsweetened shredded coconut, coconut oil, sweetener, and vanilla extract in a separate dish. Stir until it is well blended.

Stir in the pecans gently.

Using parchment paper, line a baking sheet.

Pour the mixture into the baking pan lined with parchment paper and spread uniformly. It should be about a third of an inch thick.

Bake for 40-45 minutes, or until golden brown around the edges.

Enable to cool completely in the pan before cutting and serving.

26
KETO BUFFALO CHICKEN DIP

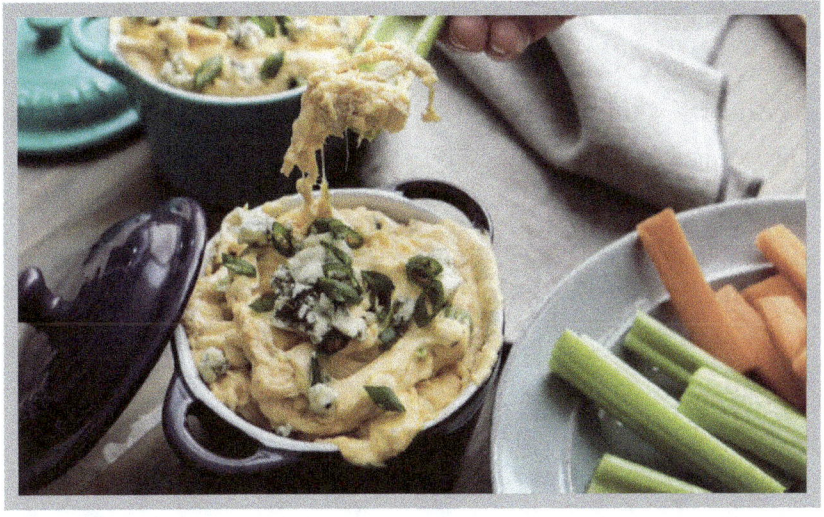

20 MINUTES

Servings 6

. . .

INGREDIENTS

- 16 ounce rotisserie chicken, shredded
- 8 ounces cream cheese, cubed
- 1 cup mozzarella cheese, shredded
- 1/3 cup buffalo hot sauce, like Frank's
- 1/2 cup ranch dressing, like Ken's
- 1 medium jalapeno, diced
- 1/4 cup green onion, chopped

PREPARATION

All ingredients should be gathered and prepared.

Melt cream cheese and mozzarella cheese together in a pan over medium-low heat.

Add the buffalo hot sauce and shredded chicken after the cheese has been thoroughly combined. To mix, stir all together thoroughly.

Combine the ranch dressing, jalapeo, and half of the green onion in a mixing bowl. Remix until it is well blended.

Cook, stirring regularly, until the mixture is hot. Serve in a warm-to-the-touch insulated serving bowl. Top with the remaining green onion and blue cheese crumbles, if desired.

To dip, serve with keto-friendly side dishes.

27
KETO CARNITAS

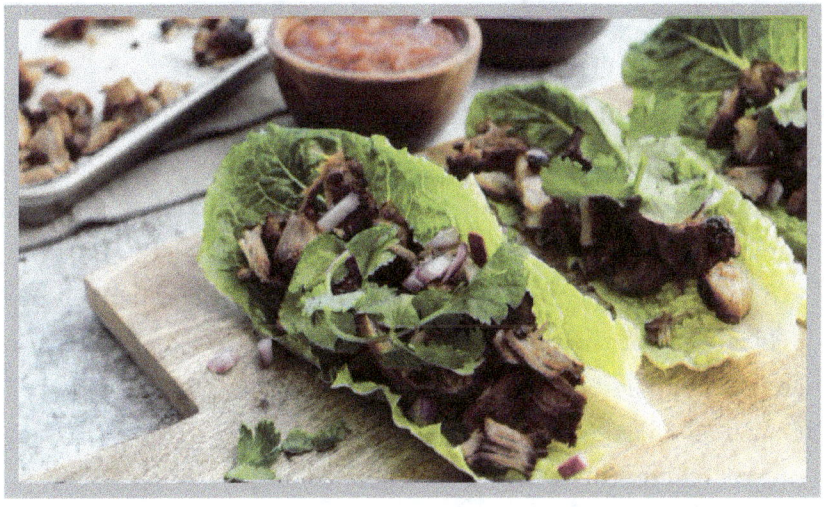

6 HOURS, 30 minutes
Servings 8

INGREDIENTS

36 ounce pork shoulder
2 tablespoon olive oil
1 tablespoon kosher salt
1/2 teaspoon black pepper
1 cup chicken broth
2 medium limes
1 medium jalapeno, seeded and diced
1 medium red onion, diced
3 cloves garlic, minced
1 teaspoon smoked paprika
1 teaspoon dried parsley
1 teaspoon dried oregano
1 teaspoon ground cumin

PREPARATION

Assemble through all the ingredients and make any appropriate preparations.

Dry the meat with paper towels before slicing it into big cubes.

Set aside the meat after seasoning it with salt and pepper.

Heat half of the olive oil in a pan over high heat. When the pan is heated, add the pork cubes and sear them for 3-4 minutes, or until all sides are browned. [Note: If you're using an Instant Pot, you can do this with the Saute function.]

Work in small batches to avoid overcrowding the pan. Keep on with the process until all of the pork has been used.

Transfer the pork to a slow cooker, then add the remaining ingredients, juicing the limes over the pork and seasoning with additional salt as required.

To ensure that all of the ingredients are uniformly distributed, stir them together.

Cook for 6 hours on low in the slow cooker. [Note: If using an Instant Pot, use the 'Meat' feature and cook for 30 minutes. After you've done, let the pressure out naturally (for around 15 minutes).]

Place the pork on a baking sheet to cool. Broil for 3-4 minutes, until slightly browned, after gently shredding with 2 forks and spooning some of the cooking juices over the end.

As needed, serve! I recommend spooning some of the cooking mixture over the pork in whatever form you're using to eat it (lettuce wraps, homemade keto tortillas, cauliflower rice). You will continue to cook the mixture in a pan to reduce it to c

28

KETO CLOUD BREAD (OOPSIE BREAD)

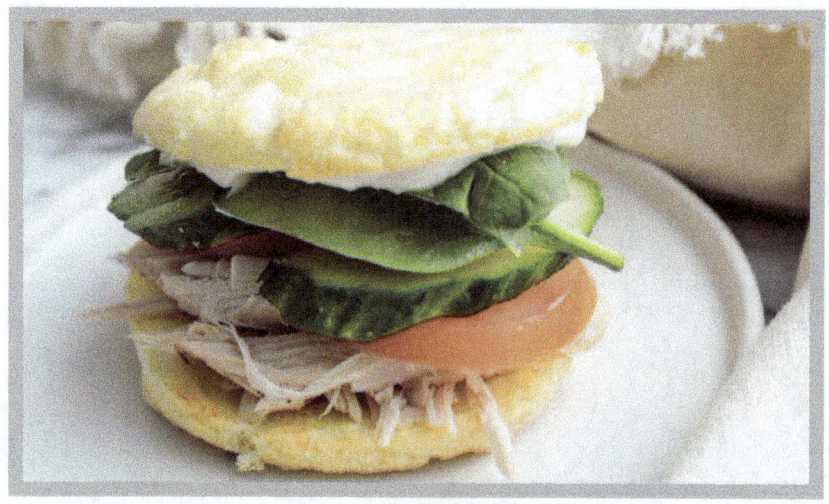

30 MINUTES

Servings 6

. . .

INGREDIENTS

- 3 large eggs, room temperature
- 1.5 ounce cream cheese, softened
- 1/8 teaspoon salt
- 1/4 teaspoon garlic powder

PREPARATION

Collect all of your ingredients. Make sure the eggs and cream cheese are both at room temperature before starting.

Preheat the oven to 300 degrees Fahrenheit. Using parchment paper, line a baking sheet.

Remove the eggs from the shells. In a large mixing bowl, whisk together the egg whites; in a smaller mixing bowl, whisk together the egg yolks.

Beat the egg whites on high speed with a hand mixer until stiff peaks develop.

Toss the egg yolks with the cream cheese, salt, and garlic. Combine these ingredients in an electric mixer and blend until smooth.

Gently fold in about a third of the egg yolk mixture into the egg whites.

After the remaining egg yolk mixture has been added, fold the egg whites together, making sure there are no white streaks in the mixture. Scoop the batter onto a baking sheet lined with parchment paper.

Spread out into a circle. The larger and flatter the cloud bread becomes, the more you extend the circle.

Preheat oven to 350°F and bake for 15-18 minutes, or until golden brown.

Enable to cool on the baking sheet for a few minutes before removing to cool completely. Use the cloud bread in every way you like (it's perfect for sandwiches and burger buns)

29
KETO TIRAMISU

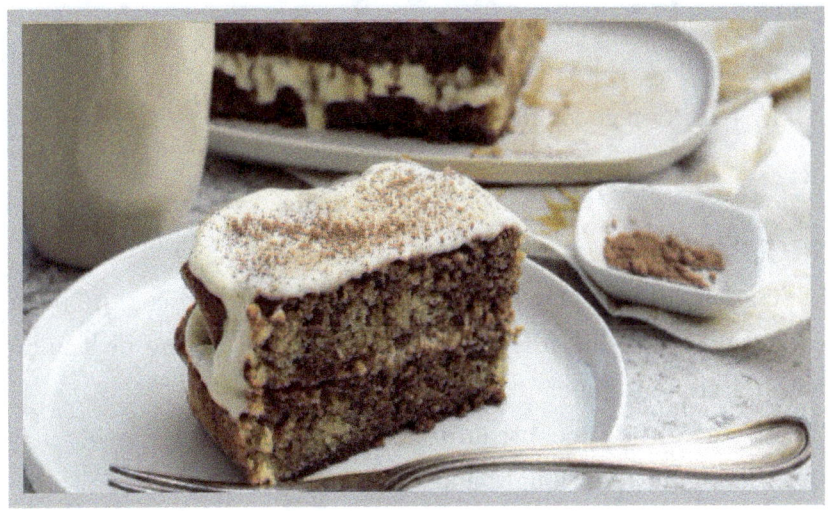

45 MINUTES
Servings 8

INGREDIENTS

Cakes

- 1/3 cup stevia/erythritol blend
- 1/3 cup butter, softened
- 3 large eggs, room temperature
- 1/4 cup heavy cream
- 1 teaspoon vanilla extract
- 1.5 cups almond flour
- 1 teaspoon baking powder
- 1 pinch sea salt
- 1/4 cup espresso or strong coffee, room temperature

Filling

- 2 large egg yolks, room temperature
- 2 tbsp. cup stevia/erythritol blend, powdered
- 4 ounce cream cheese, softened
- 1 1/2 tablespoon sour cream
- 1/2 cup heavy cream, chilled
- 1/2 teaspoon cocoa powder, for dusting

PREPARATION

Gather and prepare all of the ingredients. Preheat the oven to 350 degrees Fahrenheit. Set aside a square baking dish lined with parchment paper.

To make the cake, cream together the butter and sweetener in a mixing bowl until light and fluffy.

In a separate cup, whisk together the eggs, heavy cream, and vanilla extract.

In a separate bowl, combine the almond flour, baking powder, and salt and beat until smooth.

Move the batter to the square baking dish and smooth the

top with a spatula. Cook for 20-25 minutes, or until golden brown and a toothpick inserted in the middle comes out clean.

Begin making the filling while the cake is baking. In a metal cup, whisk together the egg yolks and powdered sweetener, then put over a pan to make a double layer. Bring the water to a boil in the tub, then reduce the heat to medium. Cook for 4-5 minutes, stirring constantly, until the egg yolk mixture is lighter in color and slightly frothy.

Remove the pan from the heat and continue to beat the mixture until it is smoother, darker in color, and smooth.

In a separate tub, whip the heavy cream until stiff peaks form.

Slowly incorporate the cream cheese and sour cream into the beaten egg yolk mixture.

Fold the cream cheese mixture into the whipped cream with a light hand.

Remove the cake from the baking dish and place it on a cutting board to cool.

Slowly pour espresso (or solid coffee) over the top of the cake until it is uniformly distributed. To make two big rectangles, cut the cake in half.

Using the filling mixture, ice one half of the cake, then put the other half on top and ice again.

Serve with a dusting of cocoa powder. Serve as a rich breakfast or a decadent dessert!

30

KETO BACON WRAPPED CHICKEN TENDERS WITH RANCH

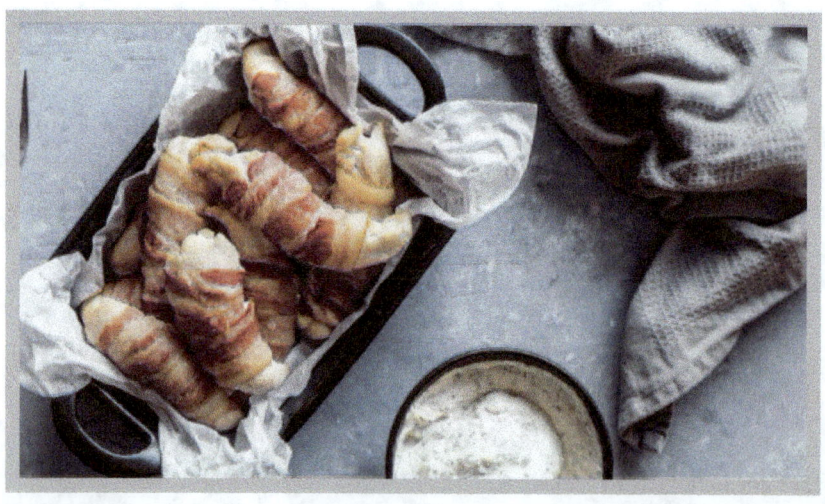

50 MINUTES
Servings 4

INGREDIENTS

- 24 ounces chicken tenders
- 10 ounces bacon
- Salt and pepper, to taste
- 1/2 cup ranch dressing

PREPARATION

Preheat oven to 400°F. Season the chicken tenders with salt and pepper before wrapping them in bacon.

Bake for 35-40 minutes, or until bacon is crisp and chicken is cooked through, on a baking sheet.

On the side, serve ranch dressing.

www.ingramcontent.com/pod-product-compliance
Lightning Source LLC
Chambersburg PA
CBHW062147100526
44589CB00014B/1723